Dirt
An Incomplete Education

By Michael Warmoth MD

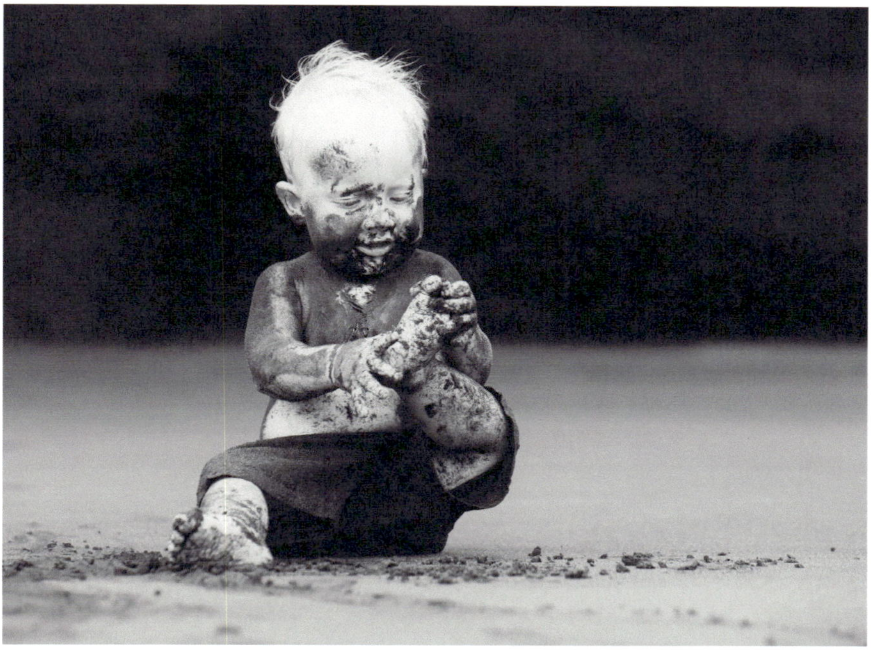

We only have so long to play in the dirt and ask questions of rivers.

-John Green

I would like to dedicate this book to
families.

Old school families that play in the dirt.
Families that persevere despite illness.

Families of all the scientists that
brought us to this summit.

Families, like the Balk Family of Grand
Rapids, that take chances to fund
aspiring researchers.

Families, like my Own, that provide
countless hours of hope and inspiration.

Families, like Crystal Brown's, who are
doggedly determined to help patients.

Families, like the Ostrowski's, who have
suffered too much because of the slow
pace of medical advances.

I. Digging in the Dirt

There is a balance in this world. Drink some water during a road race and avoid dehydration; drink too much and have your sodium level drop to the point of inducing seizures and coma. Take some acetaminophen to relieve a headache; take it too often and it may shut down your liver leaving you critically ill. Expose your child to a few kids and you'll probably educate her immune system; put her in a large daycare and it may overwhelm her and make her chronically ill.

There is an assumption that our health is solely the sum of the energy we expend and the food we eat. The right balance of each optimizes health. Maybe, in this process, we are neglecting other inputs to health. It is hard to believe that, in a world containing 5 million trillion bacteria, our health is not dependent on a partnership with these organisms.

The microbiome is a word for the collection of microorganisms which inhabit our bodies. From within our nose to the skin between our toes, from our mouths to our anuses, we have a unique combination of bacteria, yeast, and viruses which affect our health.

Plenty of incredible research is underway which examines one's microbiological 'fingerprint' and its relationship to health and disease. This fingerprint represents a current snapshot of a person and is a good place to begin. A fetus goes from having no microbiome to acquiring 100 trillion bacterial counterparts over a lifetime.

The birth canal, the breast, and sibling hands are some of the first sources of these microorganisms. Part of you may feel put-off when thinking of all this bacteria, but it's been a part of life and evolution since mammals showed up on this earth. Connections between one's microbiome fingerprint and adult conditions, such as heart disease and depression, are fascinating and pick up on the story a few decades into the process. Examining their role in the developing human is perhaps even more interesting.

We are in the middle of an unintended wide-scale experiment. The pendulum has perhaps swung too far towards cleanliness. The ubiquitous use of sanitizer, the limited amount of outdoor play, and the practice of isolating babies from siblings may be at the expense of properly educating the immune system.

Sanitation, on the other hand, is responsible for some of the greatest public health successes in history, but could an overabundance of it set us up for particular diseases, diseases which are also becoming more prominent? Is there a way to turn down the cleanliness a little without sacrificing the gains that have been made. Is there a Goldilocks level of clean, which is just right?

Back in the day, when you were a fetus, your immune system was teaching itself not to attack your own tissues (SELF) and, at the same time, to attack what was foreign (OTHERS). This differentiation between SELF and OTHERS is critical to life. Evolution did not favor those who failed this lesson.

It is becoming apparent that being born is not the end of this education but a graduation to the next level of learning. At this stage, we adopt the challenge of not only tolerating our own bodies but also incorporating the environment all around us as SELF.

It is not clear when, during a child's lifetime, the inventory marking things as SELF or OTHER is finished. It is after this point that the body knows to fight OTHERS. Recent research has shown that babies can accept organs for transplantation which are not a match; something that would be quickly rejected in an older person. The newborn is open to accept as SELF most all exposures before an unspecified age.

New recommendations have come out in regards to peanut allergy which highlight this as well. It was felt for decades that keeping children from their first exposure to peanuts, initially until age 1 and then later age 3, would protect them from peanut allergy.

Recent examination of the data reveals the exact opposite. Early exposure to peanut products protects kids from this allergy. Recommendations have changed.

This leads us to the most important message of this book:

TOLERANCE REQUIRES CONSTANT AND UBIQUITOUS EXPOSURE

It means that exposure needs to be throughout one's environment and somewhat constant over time. Incomplete or interrupted exposure results in the immune system either never knowing or forgetting what is SELF. It's like having a new bouncer at a club who doesn't recognize you because 1)You've never been there or 2) You haven't been there in a couple months.

Your immune system can 'forget' what it had previously tolerated. Many people who move back to their home state after being away for years can have new environmental allergies that they weren't expecting. I have personally noticed that a once yearly trip to Mexico from

Michigan resulted in no allergies the first time there. This is when my immune system decided the environment was OTHER and quietly built an army to fight it. The immune system usually marches into battle after a couple weeks of basic training.

My second trip was full of allergies due to my army which was at the ready. Trips three through seven went about the same but the last few trips have been well tolerated, presumably because my immune system has started the process of tolerating an environment that it is seeing recurrently.

It is crucial to note that it's not just people traveling to new environments whose immune systems are being challenged. There is also the matter of new environments traveling to people who are staying put. Globalization has allowed coffee from far away lands, tobacco from unique areas and marijuana from parts unknown to be distributed amongst areas which were usually self contained. It is within this framework of understanding that new insights and potential cures for diseases can be discovered.

Medical terminology has the tendency to distance people because of its big words and assumed complexity. We will dive into some diseases, given the simple framework we have discussed, and you will learn a good deal of knowledge without knowing any biochemistry. We will start with Multiple Sclerosis.

Multiple Sclerosis- If you've ever had an old computer or phone charger and thought- I'm not sure if these exposed wires are a good sign- then you can understand the basics of Multiple Sclerosis. Just as wires without insulation can ruin computers and phones, they can also ruin one's brain.

The immune system chews away at what it perceives to be OTHER, brain insulation. What went wrong? Why would the immune system flip the switch from SELF to OTHER?

Two things are needed to flip the switches causing the diseases mentioned in this book.

1) **A susceptible person**
2) **An environmental exposure(s)**

A susceptible person in the case of MS is one who has a unique genetic make-up and, oddly, one who has experienced infection with the Mononucleosis or the Mono virus (EBV). These people now have a unique army that is ready to battle OTHERs. This army's weak spot is that they can't distinguish between a certain bacteria and insulation, so when they see one they attack both, BUT if they are familiar with this bacteria from childhood they will stop themselves.

Let's see how this fits.

MS occurs first in teens and younger adults- This corresponds with the need for a Mono (EBV) infection as a condition for attack.

In the US, MS occurs more in the North than the South- Childhood exposure to this bacteria is higher in the South. If a susceptible person from the South encounters the bacteria in question it will *consider* an attack, but remember it is SELF and stand down. Conversely, a similar Northern child would clearly see this as OTHER and mount an attack (against the bacteria and cause collateral damage to the insulation).

Initial MS and recurrences are associated with smoking- Here is an example of the environment traveling to the individual. The bacteria in question, known to be found on tobacco leaves on occasion, is brought to the mouth of the susceptible person. Each MS flare can be thought of as the immune system boosting effect from repeated bacterial exposure.

We will give this bacteria a name, and a nickname. The name of this bacterium is Mycobacterium avium or M. Avium, and its nickname in this book is Agent Z. In fact here is a list of the usual suspects that we will refer to in the book.

Agent Z- Mycobacteria avium

Agent Y- Chlamydia pneumoniae

Agent X- Campylobacter jejuni

Our aim is to relay concepts and not get hung up on pronouncing large words.

Type I Diabetes- Let's put our knowledge to work on another disease, Type I Diabetes. It is remarkably similar to MS when examined under the microscope, except we change the target from nerve insulation to a cell which makes insulin. This cell resides in the pancreas, which spans the top of your abdomen but is towards the back. Insulin acts to keep your blood sugar down after meals and at rest. If its production is targeted, then blood sugars rise and tiny blood vessels clog. Vessels in the eyes, kidneys, feet and heart can particularly be affected.

What if Agent Z caused MS in some people, but caused Type I diabetes in others? There is evidence to support this. Perhaps, a susceptible person in the case of diabetes doesn't require the mono infection as a necessary precondition. We would then expect Type I Diabetes to occur at a younger age, which it does. There are a couple remote islands where neither MS nor Type I Diabetes existed prior to the introduction of Agent Z infected livestock.

Early exposure did not happen on these islands. An army to OTHERS resulted in any susceptible person. Rates for each of these are higher in these regions, because no one had the opportunity to educate their immune system as a young child.

In the case of Type I Diabetics, their armies can't distinguish between Agent Z and Islet Cells in the pancreas. When they see one ,they attack both.

Let's see how this fits

Type I Diabetes peaks in children between ages four and six. Agent Z causes a known benign lymph node infection in children four to six years old. - The two are not linked clinically but this shows how an age of susceptibility could be used as a clue.

Type I Diabetes in mice can be reversed with a vaccine that targets Agent Z's family.- BCG is the vaccine's name and not only has it shown promise in animal models, but it is being studied in diabetic humans by Dr. Denise Faustman at Harvard.

Mouse models for Type I Diabetes 'coincidentally' are prone to infection by the Agent Z family- NOD mice are their name and perhaps this model works for Type I diabetes precisely because of an inability to fight this unique bacterial infection.

Illustrating how the same infection might cause multiple different diseases seems important at this point. We are all unique individuals. Our cells are unique, even down to the proteins on their surface. We have cells which present invaders (OTHERS) to our immune system. They grasp these invaders in their hand showing some or most of the invader to an immune system cell. Different hands grasp things differently. Different grasps reveal alternate views of invaders. An immune system cell then attacks the specific thing that it saw. Unfortunately, it also attacks anything that looks similar. That includes other innocent cells.

II. Doppelgangers

Molecular Mimics

Attacking oneself happens through a process termed Molecular Mimicry, and it is not a new idea in medicine. The word rheumatic fever may sound familiar, but most people would have a hard time explaining it and most doctors have never seen it. A century ago this was quite different. It was caused by untreated Strep throat. The immune system would mount an attack against Strep and then attack things in the body that looked similar. Heart valves, joints and brain circuits were all affected. Rheumatic fever serves as a great model for what is going on with many autoimmune diseases. Surprisingly, little effort has gone towards finding other disease triggers after this Strep trigger was found.

Illustrated below are known and suspected mimics. An immune system cell, a T -Cell, looks at the structure of what is shown, the non-shaded part of the icon, and commits it to memory. It then attacks all things that have that exact appearance. This results in the clearance of the organism from the body AND collateral damage.

Rheumatic Fever

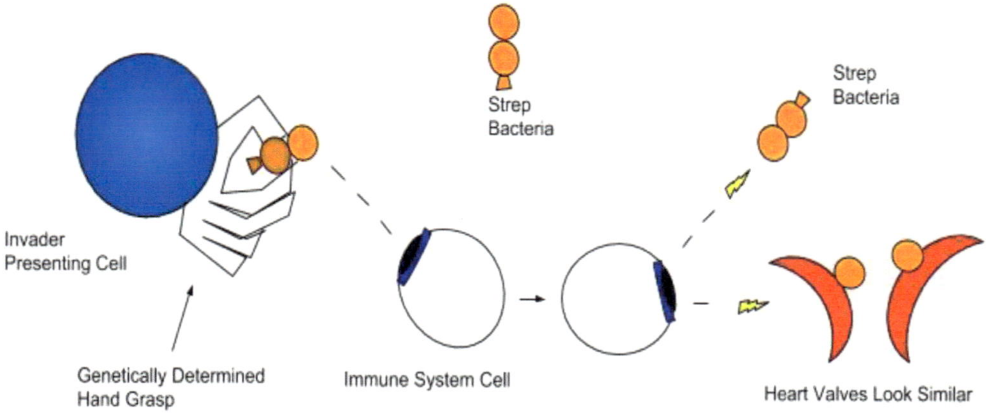

Multiple Sclerosis

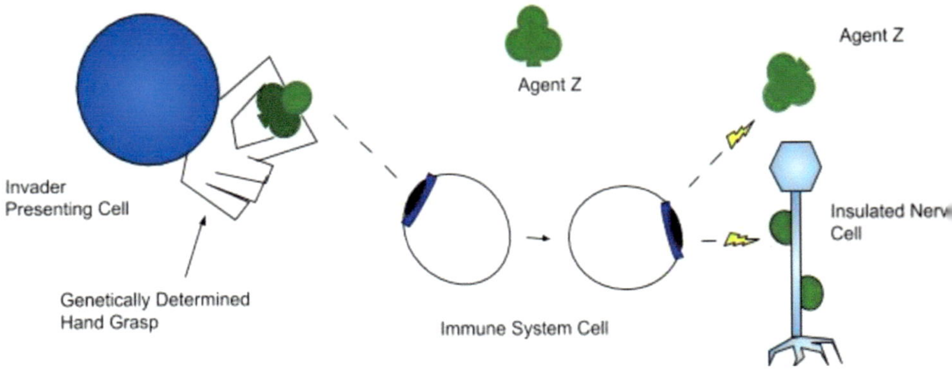

Type I Diabetes

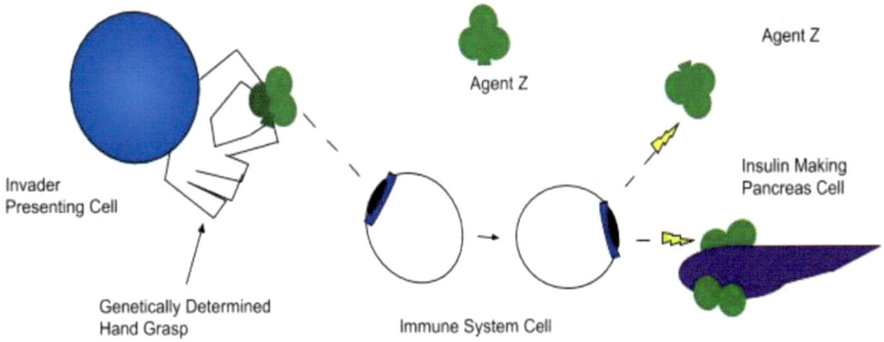

Crohn's Disease

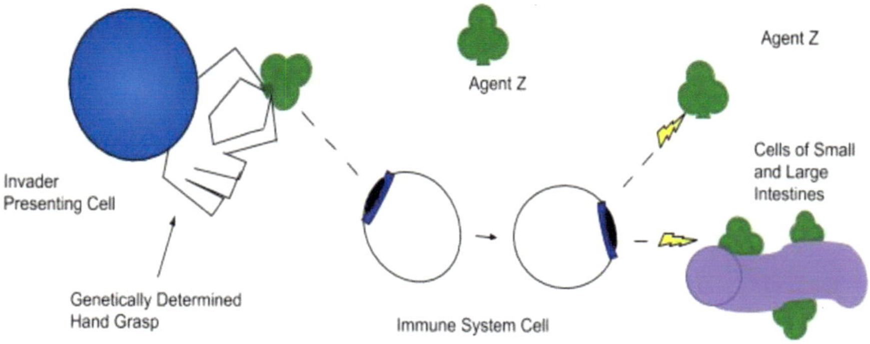

Yes, a new disease has been added, but, at this point it is easy to see the pattern- only the presenting hand and target tissue change.

If you're interested in learning more- the presenting hand is known as the MHC II (Major Histocompatibility Complex) and the eyeball is a T Cell using its TCR (T Cell Receptor) to interface with the MHC complex.

How does Crohn's disease fit into the Dirt (hygiene) Hypothesis?

Crohn's Disease

The immune system of Crohn's patients have antibodies to Agent Z- This has been found in multiple studies.

DNA of Agent Z can be found Crohn's Patients

Agent Z causes a near identical inflammatory bowel condition in cattle- In this case, it is a specific Agent Z known as MAP and the disease is known as Johne's (Yon-eeze) disease.

Children raised on dairy farms are 50% *less* likely to develop Crohn's than the general population - Exposure early and often incorporates Agent Z as SELF rather than OTHER.

Dear Critics, Don't call it infection

The link between Crohn's disease and MAP has been reported/suspected for many decades. Dr. Michael Collins at the University of Wisconsin has been an important force in the discovery and popularization of this link. Critics have been fixated on the need to find larger numbers of organisms causing infection. The mechanism of mimicry has been largely ignored. Imagine a person extremely allergic to peanuts getting a tiny whiff of peanut dust in their nose. A massive immune reaction affecting their heart, blood vessels and lungs ensues. No one really expects to find this patient's organs full of peanut dust. It's not the bulk effect of peanut dust, but rather the patient's immune system which is responsible for the damage. It's not Agent Z, Y, or X causing overwhelming infection, it's the body's reaction to each.

It is akin to finding the match that burned down the entire forest.

Identify the Culprit/Neutralize the Threat

Pinning autoimmune diseases such as MS, Type I Diabetes, and Crohn's disease on an infectious agent would be an unusual stroke of luck. This may sound odd, but it now allows us to make use of some of medicine's greatest advances. Immunization and judicious antibiotic use are responsible for saving millions of lives and will likely play a role in preventing and reversing these diseases.

If a bacteria is to blame then three treatment options emerge: Antibiotics, Targeted Vaccination, and Environmental Steps to decrease exposure to the bacteria.

i) Antibiotics seem like a good idea given how debilitating these diseases can be but there are a couple of problems. The first problem is that infections often begin without symptoms, so one would never know when to start them and the devastation due to mimicry may already be in motion. One could remain on them continuously, but the risk of bacterial resistance to the antibiotic would need to be strongly considered. Second, there are only a couple of antibiotics that work well against Agent Z and their long term use and toxicity would need to be assessed as well.

ii) Targeted vaccination is quite attractive. Blood tests could be done which would let someone know if their baseline risk has jumped from 1 in a thousand to perhaps 1 in 2. The combination of the most at risk "hand grasp" (Genetically determined MHC) and the most exuberant reaction to the mono virus/EBV (as measured by a specific antibody level) increase risk of MS by 24x and 36x respectively. Dr. Ascherio and others at Harvard are responsible for this remarkable finding. Knowing one's risk is high would make them a great candidate for a vaccine. Dr. Adel Talaat at the University of Wisconsin and Dr. Yung-Fu Chang at Cornell are leading the way with vaccines against Agent Z. A bacteria which affects livestock to a great degree.

iii) Environmental steps to decrease Agent Z, for example, would also require reaching out to the Veterinary community. The presence of this bacteria in cattle coupled with a positive association with human disease would be a call to action. Securing the safety of the milk supply from these and other mammals would become vitally important. Pasteurization has even proven inadequate to keep these organisms out of the milk supply.

Testing tobacco and Marijuana for these bacteria may be important moving forward as well, as they can contain Agent Z. This bacteria can also be found in biofilms, which are collections of bacteria and organic compounds in municipal water supplies. Researchers at the University of Illinois and other places are inventing unique ways to break up these biofilms.

III. The Other Usual Suspects

Agent X

One attribute about Agent Z is that it is clever and hides out inside cells, as opposed to bacteria like Strep which is found outside the cell. It is not the only Agent to master this strategy. Agent X (Chlamydia pneumoniae) is adept at this as well, and has been linked to the more aggressive form of Multiple Sclerosis. About 20% of MS marches forward without any significant improvement in symptoms. It is devastating to patients and their families. The two different forms of MS might be due to two different intracellular bacteria; Agent Z causing Relapsing Remitting MS (RRMS) and Agent X causing Primary Progressive MS (PPMS).

Most everyone shows evidence of infection by Agent X, often without symptoms, by age 20. People tend to get recurrent infections with

Agent X over a lifetime without even realizing it. Links to Asthma and Heart Disease have been suggested by researchers. Unlike Agent Z, it is found to be spread person to person.

East Germany and West Germany have an interesting recent past. East Germany had more air pollution and a roughly equal amounts of sunlight as compared to West Germany. The genetic history of both countries are identical.

You might expect more Asthma in East Germany, but that's not the case. Prior to the wall coming down and the reunification of Germany in the 1980's, East Germany's incidence of asthma was much lower than its neighbor. A difference which is now evaporating with the modernization of East Germany. There seems to be an asthma prevention benefit for children living in relatively impoverished, close-quarters. Perhaps they're passing around Agent X at a younger age, a more tolerant age.

Agent X deserves more study in relation to asthma development. Its DNA footprint can be found in patients with asthma flares. Could it be that a prenatal exposure is what's needed to keep the immune system from reacting to the bacteria as OTHER? Could it be that a viral infection such as RSV primes the immune system to be overly aggressive when it encounters Agent X? Stay tuned.

As mentioned previously, our model of changing the hand grasp and changing the target tissue can prove quite useful. Juvenile Rheumatoid Arthritis (now called Juvenile Idiopathic Arthritis) is a disease of childhood that not only results in swollen, hot, joints but can also lead to blindness. The immune system in these kids attacks the front of their eyes as well as the lining of their joints. Agent X has indeed been found lurking in these joints on occasion as well. It is never in numbers so great that it would be termed an infection, but it certainly seems that it may incite violence.

Agent Y

When considering MS, we saw that an attack on the insulation around nerves can be devastating to the **central** nervous system. Agent Y (Campylobacter jejuni) can provoke a very similar attack on the insulation of the **peripheral** nervous system-the nerves that run from the spinal cord to your muscles. It goes by the name Guillain-Barre (gee-yan buh-ray) Syndrome and it is likely the result of molecular mimicry between Agent Y, which causes a diarrheal illness , and those peripheral nerves. An outbreak of Agent Y results in a lot of diarrhea and a significant increase in Guillain-Barre.

The destruction of peripheral nerve function is not isolated to Guillain-Barre, it can also be seen in ALS.

Remember the Ice Bucket Challenge? It was the internet craze a few years ago that challenged people to douse themselves with freezing cold water and then nominate friends to do the same. This genius marketing idea raised millions for much needed research into one of life's most destructive diseases- ALS (Amyotrophic Lateral Sclerosis).

It is a disease where one slowly loses all motor control of their body. Walking, talking, moving and breathing all degenerate with time. Glial cells are the support system for the peripheral motor nerves. They are like a pit crew- allowing for proper functioning of the racing signals coming down the nerves. If the pit crew gets eliminated, it is only a matter of time before the nerves stop functioning. There is evidence of immune system attack amongst these glial cells in ALS.

The highest rate of diarrheal infections in the world due Agent Y is in New Zealand and this corresponds to one of the highest rates of ALS reported as well.

IV. Islands and Umbrellas

The Islands

There is a recurrent theme when investigating many of these diseases and Agents. A few islands get their unfair share of these diseases; The Faroe Islands just North of the UK, New Zealand just Southeast of Australia, and Sardinia in the Mediterranean. The first two islands were relatively free of these autoimmune diseases before colonization by the UK. The influx of livestock, and with them Agents Y and Z, may possibly have set them up for these illnesses. The older population had no chance to establish these bacteria as SELF and tolerate them. Therefore all susceptible people viewed these as OTHERs and attacked, causing the collateral damage we discussed.

In the Faroe Islands, the Multiple Sclerosis risk was much higher in anyone older than 15 years when the occupying force first arrived. Those younger than 15 apparently still had a chance to inventory the new organisms as SELF. Also, there were essentially no known cases of Crohn's or Multiple Sclerosis prior to the occupation.

In New Zealand, the rates of ALS, Crohn's and Multiple Sclerosis are all quite high. The North Island (NI) has a large cattle population, whereas the South Island (SI) has a larger sheep population. Agent Z infection of sheep is roughly double the rate of infection of cattle and thus may explain why the risk of MS is triple per capita on the SI as compared to the NI.

Sardinia has been the focus of great research by Dr. Sechi and Dr. Cossu of Italy. They have found antibody levels against Agent Z to be significantly elevated in both Type I Diabetics and MS patients.

Do umbrellas cause rain? Association vs. Causation

Umbrellas and low pressure systems moving into a region are both associated with rain, but only one of them is a cause. To date, the criticism of all of these associations is that none of them proves causation. Because of this, you may not have heard about any of these discoveries.

In the late 1800s and throughout the 1900s it was felt that for an organism to cause disease it had to adhere to a set of rules. These rules were called Koch's Postulates. The rules served us well for a while but the more we learn about cellular biology, the less relevant they've become.

Koch's Postulates

Rule 1: A human, once exposed to the organism, will develop the disease in all cases.

Poliovirus infection has shown us that only a small number will develop paralysis, while most will have mild or asymptomatic illness.

Rule 2: The human can then have the organism grown from them.

Agents Z and X are notorious for growing very poorly outside the body. Even Hepatitis B, which we know to cause cirrhosis and liver failure fails this growth stipulation.

Rule 3: Injection of the cultured organism into another person would cause the disease.

Quite unethical.

Rule 4: The organism can again be grown from the new host.

See Rule 2 exception.

One way to prove causation when dealing with these unique organisms is to vaccinate against the Agent OR encourage low-grade ongoing exposure to a weaker strain of the organism from a young age. This would allow a person or animal the ability to repel the bacteria OR recognize the bacteria as SELF and not let an overactive immune system cause tissue damage.

Agents X,Y, and Z seem like a very limited amount of bacteria to consider. There are two reasons why this is our approach. First, that's where the evidence pointed-they are the best match for the conditions being considered. Second, there are vaccines that exist for each of these disorders (in the Veterinary Medicine field) ! The veterinary community is full of brilliant minds with great knowledge of disease. Their knowledge covers more breadth than I will ever hope to acquire.

Testing mouse models of autoimmune diseases with vaccines against these Agents is a crucial step in proving causation.

As mentioned earlier, proving causation would unlock treatments such as antibiotics, vaccination and environmental control. Another therapy, which seems perfectly suited to induce tolerance, would be SubLingual ImmunoTherapy (SLIT). This has proven to be a major breakthrough in peanut allergy and I feel will deliver dramatic results in treating autoimmune disease. It involves very low doses of the inactivated bacteria of interest. The low doses are ramped up very slowly and delivered in drops that one puts under their tongue. It allows the body to view this as SELF again and orchestrate a cascade of events which will result in tolerance.

V. Flowers Rising from the Dirt

Let's Get Our Hands Dirty!

The first experiment to examine causation via vaccination has been completed. It involved a vaccine against Agent Z and a mouse model of MS known as EAE (Experimental Autoimmune Encephalitis). It was funded through the generosity of the Jim and Shirley Balk Family in Grand Rapids, Michigan. It showed that one dose of vaccine *before* the mouse ever received a disease-inducing cocktail, decreased the disability of MS by 40%. Perhaps with one booster, we could have done even better! (See Appendix A)

Getting down to work in curing these diseases can not happen fast enough. What has been presented is an organized approach to screening for autoimmune disease triggers. The cost is miniscule compared with the other research that is underway. Imagine a spreadsheet with just 3 rows, labeled Agent X,Y, and Z. The columns across the top would represent diseases that have existing mouse models. Using existing vaccines, we would try to prevent disease in these mice.

If this proves successful, we may have simultaneously found a cause and a cure. (Figure 1)

(Figure 1)

	Multiple Sclerosis	Type I Diabetes	Crohn's	Juv. Rheumatoid Arthr	Etc.
Agent Z	👍				
Agent Y					
Agent X					

Vaccination 2.0

It stands to reason that vaccines are a great preventative strategy, but many disease sufferers may feel that they are excluded from these potential advances because they're already affected. The body exists in a constant battle between injury and repair. Imagine the cells in the pancreas striving to multiply and increase their insulin production or cells which produce insulation in the brain working overtime to keep up. Could it be that recurrent exposure to Agent Z provides too much strength to the destructive side of the equation? Would inducing tolerance to Agent Z, or providing a vaccine against it, lead to a win for the repair side of the equation.

This is seeming less like a hypothetical question as the research begins to roll in. Mentioned previously, one crude vaccine against Agent Z has been shown to **reverse** Type I Diabetes in mice, and human trials are underway. Revealed in another study-The number of brain lesions in MS patients was found to **decrease** significantly after the same vaccine (BCG) was given. Both are examples of vaccinating those already affected.

No data really supports that the BCG bacteria is linked to autoimmune diseases. *But* BCG is in the same family as Agent Z, and likely provides some cross-protection to it. It is similar to shooting a shotgun at a target in the distance. The shot scatters and usually hits the bullseye and everything else. It would be much smarter to shoot at our target with a precision rifle. That is the goal. A vaccine targeted specifically towards our *Agent* of interest so that it hits the target every time.

Lastly, more evidence of the effectiveness of late vaccination can be seen in a disease known as Dengue Fever. It is a viral, flu-like illness which can progress to diffuse spontaneous bleeding. This doesn't typically occur with one's first infection but rather one's second.

When developing the vaccine, it became evident that vaccinating Dengue 'Virgins' merely primed them to get hit harder when they caught it the **second** time in the community BUT vaccinating the '**once-infected**' was key to preventing severe disease.

Mimicry: The Sequel

Delving into these three bacteria, excluding all other organisms, may seem to represent too narrow a focus. It is a good start based on the available evidence.

We have seen that bacteria may resemble human cells, so it seems reasonable that bacteria may resemble other bacteria and viruses as well. For the Mathematicians and Philosophers out there- If A causes C and B looks like A, perhaps B causes C as well.

It has been my experience with a few patients, and is now a large-scale study, that the virus that causes Hand, Foot and Mouth disease (Coxsackie Virus) may be responsible for some cases of Type I Diabetes. I suspect that Agent Z and Coxsackie Virus share some structural similarities.

Can you imagine how utilizing Big Data to catalog the 3D structure of organisms and comparing them to each other could accelerate this type of research? Find a triggering organism, then find its look-alikes.

So many diseases, so little time!

We have just expanded the number of organisms that may trigger the above mentioned diseases. Now it's time to touch on diseases not yet mentioned.

Acute Lymphoblastic Leukemia (A.L.L.) in Children-Agent Z and A.L.L. peak infection age are the same. Data in frogs revealed a leukemia-like condition due to an Agent Z family member.

Hashimoto's Thyroid Disease- Similar to A.L.L. in its distribution. It's felt in some circles that once a cause for A.L.L. is found, this will also be the cause of Hashimoto's.

Schizophrenia - This disease shares some similarities with MS when it comes down to age and geographical distribution. Fascinating research has tied a bacteria known as Toxoplasma (Toxo) to Schizophrenia. It is similar to Agent Z in that it too hides within cells and can inhabit the environment. One limitation with Toxo is the typical need for cats in the life cycle. Given this, it may be that both bacteria are important and act through a similar mechanism- as not all cases of Schizophrenia can be linked to cat owners.

In her book *Brain on Fire*, Susannah Cahalan describes her descent into mental illness and presumed schizophrenia and how, thanks to her own courage and proximity to brilliant scientists, she was able to recognize it as a specific autoimmune phenomenon. What if mental illnesses such as depression, schizophrenia, and obsessive compulsive disorder were all the result of antibodies against perceived OTHERS which then affected brain functioning. It would further reinforce the need to recognize the intense biological pathology that afflicts those with mental illnesses.

In his book, *Hidden Valley Road*, Robert Kolker details a family devastated by Schizophrenia affecting many of its children. Genetic studies pinpointed a mutated SHANK2 gene. The associated protein is critical for relaying signals in the brain. The SHANK2 mutation is often associated with a CHRNA7 mutation and *this* mutation is associated with 1) Poor brain signaling AND 2) Susceptibility to the Agent Z family.

Sarcoidosis-This is a disease that causes lesions in the lungs, hearts and other organs. These lesions resemble the ones caused by Agent Z family members: Tuberculosis and Leprosy. The suspicion that Agent Z is involved is nothing new but,in light of the specific vaccines that we are proposing, likely warrants another look. When you talk about allergy, some people just have a low grade chronic problem rather than any dramatic reaction. This is true for those who may find themselves tolerating a pet because the family is in love with that dog. For unknown reasons, they remain stuck between full tolerance and profound reaction. It could be that Sarcoid results from a low grade reaction chronically to repeated Agent Z exposure over the years.

Breast Cancer- The stats behind some breast cancers are remarkably similar to Multiple Sclerosis. This is not to say that they are related, but may be accelerated by similar circumstances. Data from New Zealand show an acceleration in risk between the ages 20-40 but a slower rise after age 40, similar to MS. EBV infection as a primer has been a suggestion in regards to Breast Cancer as well as with MS.

Dorothy Rybacyzk Pathak Ph.D. at Michigan State University has studied the Polish populations in the Midwest and their Breast Cancer risk. The goes up dramatically once a family immigrates here. Oddly, it appears that adherence to the old country's diet is a protective factor against Breast Cancer. Sauerkraut-eating adolescents have a 72% less risk of later developing Breast Cancer. Certainly, this has sparked an interest into the chemical properties of the food but maybe we should take a broader look as well.

What is Sauerkraut? Cabbage+Bacteria+Salt+ Time When viewed through our "Dirt" perspective, could constant and ubiquitous Sauerkraut and its bacterial components act as a way to immunotolerate other environmental bacterial triggers.

Melanoma- There is an odd couple of clusters of a rare melanomas (uveal melanoma) that may interest you. Cracking this case may provide clues to how standard melanoma spreads and may open new avenues to treatment.

Melanoma is a cancer of a pigmented skin cell and can also occur within the eye. As reported by Orloff et. al. at Thomas Jefferson University, 3 college roommates in Alabama developed melanoma in the front part of their eye 10-20 years after leaving college and 5 kids from a high school in North Carolina did the same.

In 1982, another cluster of 3 in a small community was found. In this case, Dr. Louria of Newark N.J. exposed mice to the same water after they were weaned from their mothers and found that 9 of 60 developed eye growths whereas none of the controls (0 of 30; those exposed to "safe" water) were affected.

Bacteria living in water systems can congregate anywhere- from the supply line into the building to a single showerhead. Agent Z outbreaks have occurred via showerheads. Legionella is a bacteria that got its very name by colonizing a cooling tower for the air conditioning in a hotel hosting an American Legion Convention. This resulted in hundreds of hospitalizations and 29 deaths. Legionella usually causes significant symptoms in only a couple percent of people, leaving it free to covertly act as an another Agent (Agent L?). Clusters that share the same water supply should not only look at the chemicals in the water, but also try to grow the bacteria from these pipes and ducts as well.

ALS/Parkinson's- It may seem odd to put these in the same category, but there is a curious story about the epidemiology of each: a co-clustering event in the 1950's in the Western Pacific Ocean. Similar to the Faroe Islands' introduction of Agent Z by an occupying force, this involves another Axis member. The Japanese occupied Guam and other nearby islands during World War II. A live Japanese fish was introduced to these islands. This fish carried an asymptomatic infection of an Agent Z family member; Mycobacterium marinum. Many locals developed a skin infection from this bacteria, known at the time as 'SPAM' , from bathing in this water.

Similar to the British occupying force in the Faroe Islands:

1) Occupier introduces Mycobacterial Species (Agent Z)
2) 10-15 year lag in time
3) Chronic Inflammatory Disease

Faroe Islands=> MS and Crohn's

Guam=> ALS and Parkinson's

One would reason that, based on this book and the concept that early exposure leads to tolerance, cases would decline as children assimilated to the environmental change.

And that is exactly what happened!

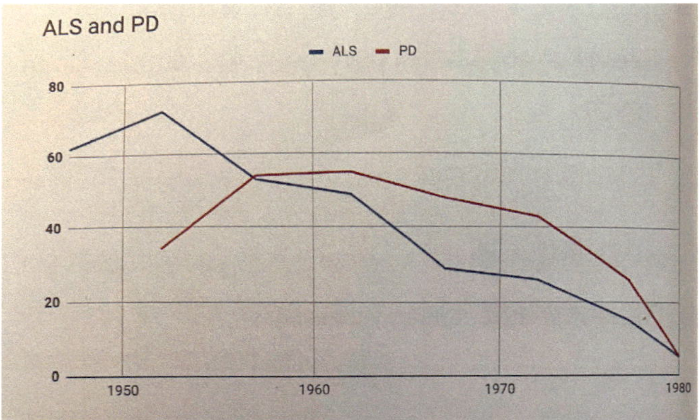

Five-Year Annual Incidence Rates per 100,000 of ALS and PD in Western Pacific Males

Steele and Guzman 1987 Canadian Journal of Neurological Sciences

Other clues to **Parkinson's** being infectiously triggered include:

1) A cluster of four people on a 1970's TV show, including Michael J Fox, who

filmed in a similar stuffy location and shared the same air and water. They developed Parkinson's disease 10-20 years later.

2) Nepal has one of the largest Parkinson's populations. Nearly everyone lives with livestock and more of that livestock is now infected with Agent Z. Perhaps Nepal could be thought of as an island atop a mountain.

A few words about the LRRK2 gene-This is a gene which predisposes some to Parkinson's and "coincidentally" predisposes to Agent Z infection.

A few words about MPTP mice- This Parkinson's mouse model benefits from Agent Z vaccination. It protects their brain.

VI. Wallflowers and Snowballs

Not Attractive Enough to Dance with Big Pharma

There is no conspiracy to date keeping these ideas from taking hold, but rather an abundance of conformity. Resistance to new ideas is ubiquitous. Below is a sample of roadblocks from drug manufacturers and disease foundations.

“We don't fund basic science.”

“We have a group of scientists that we fund year after year.”

“Why would the answer come from outside the specialty field?”

“Why would we invest in a one time vaccine when we could make money every month lessening the effects of a chronic illness?”

The current medication landscape is reactive as opposed to proactive/preventative.

Snowballs

Imagine a boy at the top of a snowy mountain range making a series of tiny snowballs. Now picture 7 small villages at the base of the mountains. He begins to roll each snowball. They all pick up speed and size until they are a legitimate threat to the towns. Big pharmaceutical companies devise strategies that reinforce these metaphorical towns with walls. Unfortunately, they can't get around to protecting more than a few towns. Wall building is expensive and, although it works for a few towns, many are devastated. This represents the focus of current pharmaceutical development. There is not an incentive to find inciting events, it is financially less lucrative for them to proceed in this direction.

Stopping the boy from making the snowballs in the first place is a far greater strategy. Finding the triggers, removing them from the environment and developing vaccines or tolerance strategies are all steps we can take to disarm the boy.

Balance is required going forward. Dismissing the gains of sanitation, vaccination and judicious antibiotic use would spell disaster. Salmonella, Botulism, Meningitis, and Flesh-Eating Bacteria would all be welcomed back in such a scenario.

On the other hand, what harm can come from a child helping in the garden and getting a little dirty. How harmful would it be to return to reasonable sized playgroups and outdoor sports now that COVID is waning in overall severity? Maybe we should return to washing hands after restroom use and before meals as opposed to constant sanitizer use.

Just as the Apollo 11 moon shot took math and science off the page and sent it hurtling through space (and back), so should these lessons of biology send us on a journey to cure multiple diseases by 2025.

APPENDIX 1:

A Model which can be replicated and refined for all of the diseases and Agents listed.

The Effect of Targeted Vaccination Against Mycobacterium Avium ssp. Paratuberculosis (MAP) in a Multiple Sclerosis Mouse Model: Implications for Causation

Michael R. Warmoth MD

Epidemiologic evidence relating to the causation of Multiple Sclerosis, based upon twin concordance studies, implicates both genetic and environmental contributions. The HLA-DRB1/ HLA-A haplotype confers a 23 fold increase in MS prevalence above its baseline of 1 per 1,000 persons. Epigenetic factors, such as an aberrant response to Epstein Barr Virus (EBV) and Vitamin D deficiency can increase that risk 36 and 2 fold respectively. Evidence of an association between elevated MAP antibodies and Multiple Sclerosis has been reported.

A prospective randomized controlled trial was performed in SJL mice exposed to the myelin-related oligopeptide $PLP_{139\text{-}151}$; a relapsing-remitting Experimental Autoimmune Encephalitis (EAE) model. 100 mice were randomized into five groups of 20. Group 1-Unimmunized prior to disease induction. Group 2- Immunized twice with a 74 kDa fusion protein vaccine against MAP; delivered 28 days and 7 days prior to disease induction. Group 3- 1 dose of 74 kDa vaccine 10 days post-disease induction. Group 4- Attenuated whole cell MAP vaccine (ΔSigH) 28 days

prior to disease induction. Group 5- ΔSigH vaccine 10 days post disease induction.
Disability was quantified using a EAE disability scoring reference ranging from 0 to 5.Significant decreases in peak disability were seen in the bimodal peaks of this relapsing-remitting model 38% ($p<0.006$) and 40% ($p<0.001$). ΔsigH immunized mice lost half as much weight as controls post disease induction. The results suggest that environmental MAP antigen exposure may play an etiologic role in the development of EAE.

Introduction

The sine qua non of Multiple Sclerosis (MS) involves immune-mediated destruction of myelin in the central nervous system resulting in scarring, abnormal conductivity, and resulting disability. There are two forms of the disease. Relapsing-remitting MS accounts for 80% of the disease burden whereas the primary progressive form accounts for 20%. Twin studies show concordance for MS between identical twins to be 30% and 3% between fraternal twins [1]. This suggests contributions from genetics as well as the environment.

Genetic evaluations have shown increased risk of MS with haplotypes HLA-A as well as HLA-DRB1, the combination of which leads to a 23 fold increase [2]. Known predisposing factors, which may work through epigenetic mechanisms, include low vitamin D levels and aberrant response to Epstein Barr Virus (EBV) infection. Vitamin D deficiency has been associated with a two fold increased risk of MS [3]. High levels of Epstein Barr Nuclear Antibody (EBNA) confer a thirty six fold increase in risk [4].

Kurtzke et.al. detailed an epidemiologic case for infection as that environmental agent [5]. Investigation of MS clusters have revealed some clues. One, in the Faroe

Islands, highlighted the rise in MS incidence years after British military occupation [5] and another, in Galion Ohio, revealed an increased MS incidence after a soil giveaway associated with a new high school gymnasium construction [5]. These suggest a possible fastidious organism, which has been further bolstered by studies associating Mycobacterium avium *ssp. paratuberculosis* with MS. Cossu et. al. reported higher humoral titers to MAP in M.S. patients [6] and Mameli et. al. reported increased serum and CSF reactivity to MAP antigens in patients as well [7]. With respect to EAE murine models, an increased genetic susceptibility to mycobacterial species has been shown [8] and mycobacterial cage contamination can be present [9].

Prior Epstein Barr Virus (EBV) has been found to be present in 100% of MS patients [10]. The high level of seroconversion of non-MS patients suggests that it is likely necessary, but not sufficient to cause Multiple Sclerosis. EBV may lay the groundwork for a second hit to occur resulting in MS. Establishing causation for a second-hit agent may be problematic if we adhere to Koch's Postulates. If, for example, the second hit induces a molecular mimicry with myelin antigens then immunologic clearance of the agent may occur leaving little trace. An alternate way of establishing causation would be to immunize against the infectious agent and see if this prevents the disease. Ristori et.al. have reported some success in treating MS with BCG [11], which may act as a crude vaccine for MAP, just as Cowpox was a crude but effective vaccine against Smallpox in the late 1700's.

We have set out to immunize against MAP specifically in EAE mice to see if this significantly decreases neurologic disability. Our findings suggest a large and significant improvement in mice which were immunized against MAP prior to disease induction.

Methods

ΔsigH vaccine preparation

A live attenuated M. avium ssp. *paratuberculosis* vaccine was prepared by Dr. Talaat's lab as described in Shippy et. al. [12]. The sigH regulator gene was altered to decrease MAP pathogenicity.

74 kDa. fusion protein preparation

The 74 kDa. fusion protein vaccine was constructed de novo at Proteos Labs (Kalamazoo, MI) from the DNA sequence provided by Dr. Chang's lab in Chen et. al. [13]

SJL mice immunization

Day -28 Cryo-vials on dry ice from Proteos containing 0.5 mg/ml Map74F in TBS, pH 7.4 received. The vaccine was stored at -80°C.

Day -22 100 SJL mice (Envigo, male, PO #193687, R #3778, 5-6 weeks old) were received, individually examined and housed in ten filter-topped cages of ten mice each in a HEPA-filtered enclosure. The mice were placed in quarantine with daily inspections.

Day -21 The mice were ear tagged (SOP 810) with unique numbers for identification purposes, and weighed (RESULTS) and sorted into five treatment groups of 20 mice each based upon average body weight.

Day -15 Received via Federal Express on coolants from the University of Wisconsin in 50 ml conical tubes and stored at 4-8°C

Day 0 Group 1: 2 ml sterile PBS (Sigma, Cat. D8537, lot RNBR3321) was added to one vial Ribi adjuvant system (RAS, Sigma, Cat. S6322, lot 125M4172V) which had been warmed to 40°C. The mixture was vortexed for 3 minutes, inverted and vortexed for an addition minute.

Group 2: RAS was warmed to 40°C prior to addition of 2 ml (2 vials) Map74F (equilibrated to room temperature).

The mixture was vortexed for 3 minutes, inverted and vortexed for an addition minute.
Group 4: 1 ml of the SigH was diluted into 1 ml sterile PBS.
The mice were weighed (RESULTS). The mice in Groups 1, 2, 4 were injected subcutaneously (SC, SOP 1610) with 0.1 ml of their respective vaccine.

Day 21

Group 1: 2 ml sterile PBS was added to one vial RAS which had been warmed to 40°C. The mixture was vortexed for 3 minutes, inverted and vortexed for an addition minute.
Group 2: RAS was warmed to 40°C prior to addition of 2 ml (2 vials) Map74F (equilibrated to room temperature). The mixture was vortexed for 3 minutes, inverted and vortexed for an addition minute. The mice were weighed (RESULTS). The mice in Groups 1, and 2 were injected SC with 0.1 ml of their respective vaccine.

Day 28 15 mg $PLP_{139\text{-}151}$ (BioSynthesis, lot T6928) was dissolved in 15 ml sterile PBS to prepare a 1 mg/ml solution. 100 mg heat-killed *Mycobacterium tuberculosis* H37 RA (Difco, Cat. 231141) was homogenized in 50 ml squalene (Sigma, Cat. S3626, lot 118K0847) to prepare a 2 mg/ml suspension (Complete Freund's Adjuvant, CFA) 50 µg pertussis toxin (Sigma, Cat. P7206, lot SLBR6905V) was dissolved in 50 ml sterile PBS to prepare a 1 µg/ml solution. 11 x [1ml PLP was homogenized with 1 ml CFA] on an ice bath. A droplet of the emulsion
floated on water did not disperse. The mice were weighed and injected SC in both flanks with 0.1 ml PLP/CFA emulsion. One hour later the mice were injected by intraperitoneal route (IP, SOP 1630) with 0.2 ml pertussis toxin (200 ng/mouse).

Day 3050 µg pertussis toxin was dissolved in 50 ml sterile PBS to prepare a 1 µg/ml solution.
The mice were injected IP with 0.2 ml pertussis toxin (200 ng/mouse).

Day 38 RAS was warmed to 40°C prior to addition of 2 ml (2 vials) Map74F (equilibrated to room temperature). The mixture was vortexed for 3 minutes, inverted and vortexed for an addition minute.

Group 5: 1 ml of the SigH was diluted into 1 ml sterile PBS.

The mice were weighed (RESULTS). The mice in Groups 3 and 5 were injected subcutaneously (SC, SOP 1610) with 0.1 ml of their respective vaccine.

Days 29-67 The mice were weighed (RESULTS) and scored daily

for signs of disease as in TABLE 1.

Table 1

TABLE 1: EAE SCORING PARAMETERS

Score	Clinical Signs
0	No obvious signs of motor dysfunction in mice compared to non-immunized control
0.5	Distal Tail Limpness
1	Limp or floppy tail
2	Limp tail and weakness in hind legs
3.	Limp tail and complete paralysis of hind legs (most common) OR Limp tail with paralysis of one front and one hind leg **OR** all of the following: - severe head tilting - walking only along the edges of the cage - pushing against the cage wall - spinning when picked up by the tail
4.	Limp tail, complete hind leg and partial front leg paralysis - Mouse is minimally moving around cage but appears alert and feeding. Euthanasia is recommended after mouse scores 4 for 2 consecutive days. A score of 5 is entered when mouse is euthanized.
5.	Complete hind and complete front leg paralysis, no movement around cage **OR** Mouse is spontaneously rolling in cage **OR** Mouse found dead due to paralysis. If mouse is alive, the mouse is euthanized immediately. A score of 5 is entered for that mouse for all days remaining in the study.

Mice may be given intermediate scores such as 1.5, 2.5 or 3.5 when the clinical picture lies between two defined scores.

Statistical Analysis

Daily disability scores were documented and significance (p-value) was calculated vs Group 1 by two-way ANOVA followed by Bonferroni post test analysis.

Results

Vaccination targeted against MAP was effective in providing significant relief from neurologic disability in the EAE mouse model of Relapsing-Remitting Multiple Sclerosis. Peak disability, as measured by the EAE Scoring Parameters, was 38% less ($p<0.006$) in the SigH immunized mice for the first flare of disability and 40% less ($p<0.001$) for the relapse (Fig. 1).

Fig.1

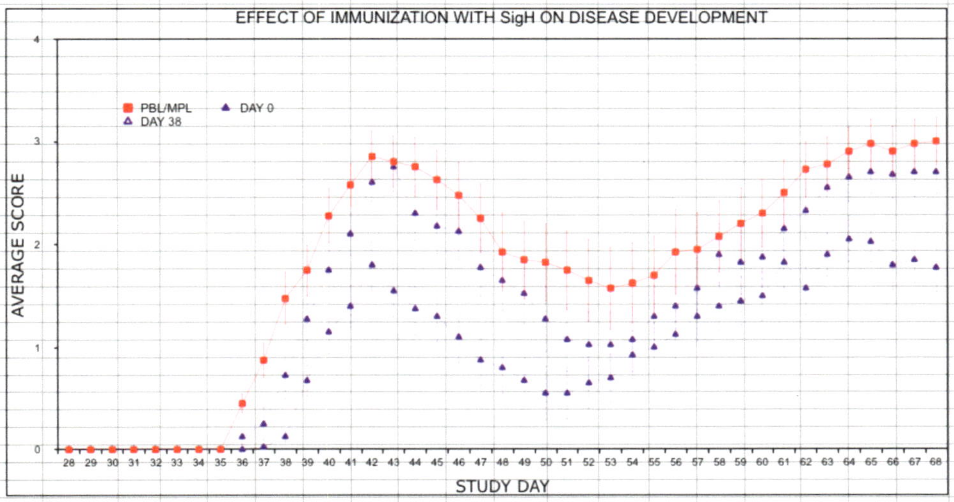

The 74 kDa Fusion vaccine resulted in a 24% reduction ($p<0.03$) in the first flare of disability and a 23% ($p<0.05$) for the relapse (Fig. 2). Late vaccination with either vaccine, once clinical disease onset occurred, did not result in statistically significant decreases in disability.

Fig.2

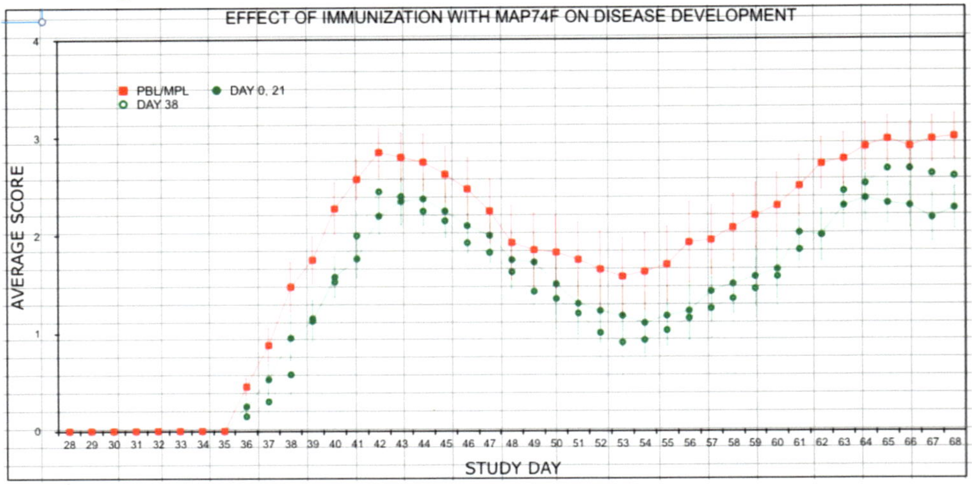

In addition to improvement in disability scores, mice immunized with the ΔsigH vaccine, either before or after disease induction, exhibited significantly less weight loss ($p< 0.05$, $p<0.05$) compared to pre-disease induction weights. -11.56% for Control Group 1, -4.5% for Group 4, and -5% for group 5. (Fig. 3)

Fig.3

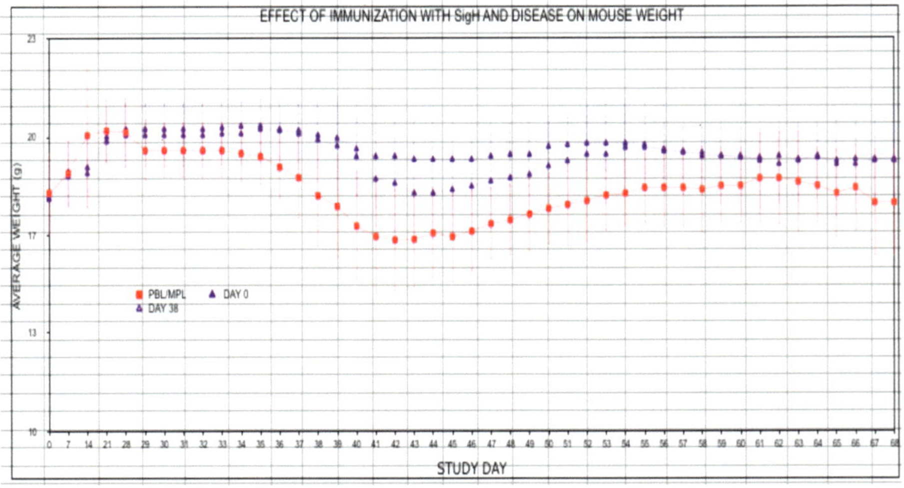

Discussion

These findings represent an evolution from examining associations between multiple sclerosis and MAP to establishing a causative role for such agents. Establishing causation results in a myriad of actionable interventions to assist those suffering from MS.

MAP's presence can be found in the dairy industry as a cause for Johne's disease, an autoimmune inflammatory intestinal condition. Widespread vaccination does not occur to date. Pasteurized milk can contain viable MAP as well as its epitopes [14]. Subsequent contamination of groundwater and soil occur with MAP, and it is represented in biofilms in municipal water supplies [15]. An effective bovine vaccination program and further research on destroying biofilms could modify the risk of developing MS or its relapses.

Focused human vaccination for susceptible individuals, those with a HLA-DRB1 haplotype and/or those with elevated EBV antibodies, would also be an option. Support is further suggested by the Ristori et. al. finding that *BCG* can decrease MS lesions on MRI. [11] Formerly thought to be a nonspecific immune system booster, *BCG* and it's mycobacterial antigens may represent partial vaccination against MAP. If EBV is considered the first hit and MAP is considered the second hit in this pathogenic mechanism, it follows that EBV vaccination efforts continue in earnest.

Apart from environmental containment efforts and vaccination, a third avenue of treatment might focus on inducing tolerance to MAP antigens at a young age. An environmental cline exists in MS epidemiology which reveals a higher risk of developing MS as distance from the equator increases.(Fig.4)

Fig. 4

World distribution of multiple sclerosis: greater prevalence in higher northern and southern latitudes

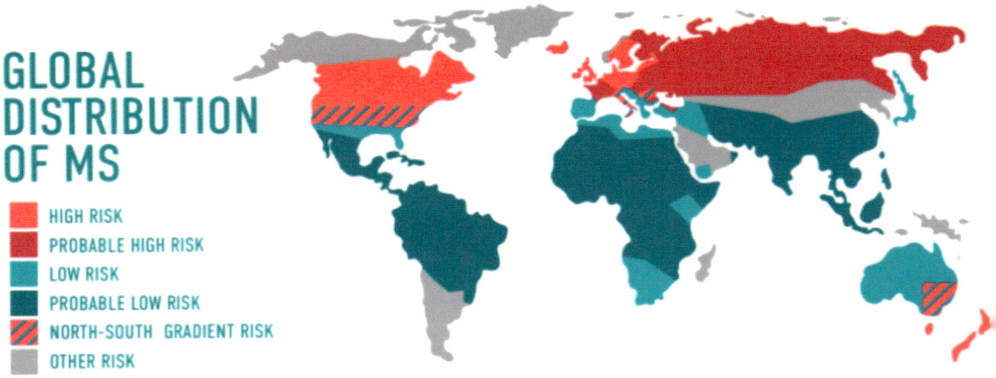

REFERENCES

Ramagopalan SV, Sadovnick AD. Genetics and epidemiology of multiple sclerosis. In Giesser BS, ed. Primer on Multiple Sclerosis. New York, NY: Oxford University Press; 2011:15-29.

It has also been shown that moving from a low-incidence area to a high-incidence area after age fifteen will result in an individual having a MS risk equivalent to that of the low-risk prior address [16,17] Whereas, an individual moving from a high to low incidence area will retain that higher risk if that person is older than fifteen. This may act as an epidemiologic clue linking EBV and MAP as the average age of seroconversion to EBV is the teen years [18]. It follows that exposure and subsequent tolerance to M. Avium prior to EBV infection may be protective whereas EBV acquisition in a susceptible individual prior to MAP exposure may be pathologic. Support for an exposure cline to match the MS disease cline can be traced to US military recruit data from the 1950's [19]. A PPD study using M.avium proteins revealed higher rates of positivity in Southern recruits (70%) relative to their Northern counterparts (20%).

Overall, these findings highlight the need to systematically investigate suspected infectious triggers for MS and other autoimmune diseases with the goal of not merely uncovering associations but making an attempt to establish causative links through vaccination. Establishing these links would open the door to antiinfectives, vaccination, and perhaps immunotherapy. All of which would get closer to prevention than the current medication options, which reflect downstream damage control and are prohibitively expensive.

Acknowledgements: Funding for this research made possible by a grant from Jim and Shirley Balk/Spectrum Health Foundation. The Agent Z Club was also instrumental in making this a reality: Crystal Brown PT, Chris Ostrowski, Eric Brown MD

1. Willer CJ, Dyment DA, Risch NJ, Sadovnick AD, Ebers GC, Canadian Collaborative Study G. Twin concordance and sibling recurrence rates in multiple sclerosis. Proc Natl Acad Sci U S A. 2003;100(22):12877-82.

2. Brynedal B, Duvefelt K, Jonasdottir G, Roos IM, Akesson E, Palmgren J, et al. HLA-A confers an HLA-DRB1 independent influence on the risk of multiple sclerosis. PLoS One. 2007;2(7):e664.

3. Mokry LE, Ross S, Ahmad OS, Forgetta V, Smith GD, Goltzman D, et al. Vitamin D and Risk of Multiple Sclerosis: A Mendelian Randomization Study. PLoS Med. 2015;12(8):e1001866.

4. Munger KL, Levin LI, O'Reilly EJ, Falk KI, Ascherio A. Anti-Epstein-Barr virus antibodies as serological markers of multiple sclerosis: a prospective study among United States military personnel. Mult Scler. 2011;17(10):1185-93.

5. Kurtzke JF. Epidemiologic evidence for multiple sclerosis as an infection. Clin Microbiol Rev. 1993;6(4):382-427.

6. Cossu D, Cocco E, Paccagnini D, Masala S, Ahmed N, Frau J, et al. Association of Mycobacterium avium subsp. paratuberculosis with multiple sclerosis in Sardinian patients. PLoS One. 2011;6(4):e18482.

7. Mameli G, Cocco E, Frau J, Marrosu MG, Sechi LA. Epstein Barr Virus and Mycobacterium avium subsp. paratuberculosis peptides are recognized in sera and cerebrospinal fluid of MS patients. Sci Rep. 2016;6:22401.

8. Chiodini RJ, Buergelt CD. Susceptibility of Balb/c, C57/B6 and C57/B10 mice to infection with Mycobacterium paratuberculosis. J Comp Pathol. 1993;109(4):309-19.

9. Kaliste E, Linnainmaa M, Meklin T, Torvinen E, Nevalainen A. The bedding of laboratory animals as a source of airborne contaminants. Lab Anim. 2004;38(1):25-37.

10. Ascherio A, Munger KL. Epstein-barr virus infection and multiple sclerosis: a review. J Neuroimmune Pharmacol. 2010;5(3):271-7.

11. Ristori G, Buzzi MG, Sabatini U, Giugni E, Bastianello S, Viselli F, et al. Use of Bacille Calmette-Guerin (BCG) in multiple sclerosis. Neurology. 1999;53(7):1588-9.

12. Shippy DC, Lemke JJ, Berry A, Nelson K, Hines ME, 2nd, Talaat AM. Superior Protection from Live-Attenuated Vaccines Directed against Johne's Disease. Clin Vaccine Immunol. 2017;24(1).

13. Chen LH, Kathaperumal K, Huang CJ, McDonough SP, Stehman S, Akey B, et al. Immune responses in mice to Mycobacterium avium subsp. paratuberculosis following vaccination with a novel 74F recombinant polyprotein. Vaccine. 2008;26(9):1253-62.

14. Chiodini RJ, Hermon-Taylor J. The thermal resistance of Mycobacterium paratuberculosis in raw milk under conditions simulating pasteurization. J Vet Diagn Invest. 1993;5(4):629-31.

15. Torvinen E, Lehtola MJ, Martikainen PJ, Miettinen IT. Survival of Mycobacterium avium in drinking water biofilms as affected by water flow velocity, availability of phosphorus, and temperature. Appl Environ Microbiol. 2007;73(19):6201-7.

16. Ascherio A, Munger KL. Environmental risk factors for multiple sclerosis. Part I: the role of infection. Ann Neurol. 2007;61(4):288-99.

17. Ascherio A, Munger KL. Environmental risk factors for multiple sclerosis. Part II: Noninfectious factors. Ann Neurol. 2007;61(6):504-13.

18. De Paschale M, Clerici P. Serological diagnosis of Epstein-Barr virus infection: Problems and solutions. World J Virol. 2012;1(1):31-43.

19. Edwards LB, Acquaviva FA, Livesay VT, Cross FW, Palmer CE. An atlas of sensitivity to tuberculin, PPD-B, and histoplasmin in the United States. Am Rev Respir Dis. 1969;99(4):Suppl:1-132.

About the Author:

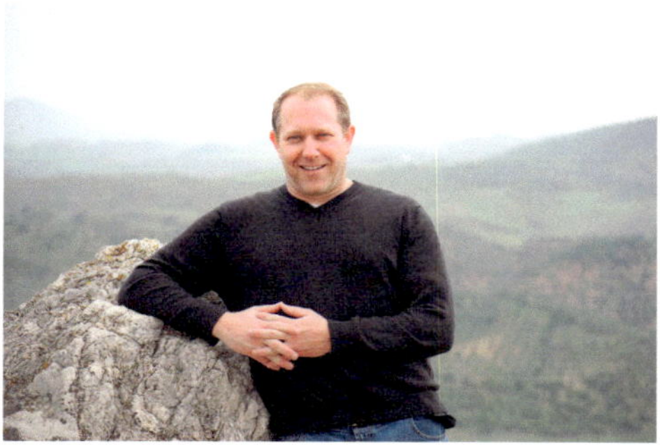

Dr. Warmoth lives in Petoskey, Michigan but has been exchanging ideas and research designs with scientists at the University of Wisconsin, Cornell University, Northwestern University, Colorado State University as well as Michigan State University.

Made in the USA
Las Vegas, NV
08 November 2026

57691396R00040